# CRACKING THE EGG

*Understanding Fertility and*

*Reproductive Health*

## JOSEPH HONESTY

# Table of Contents

# CONCLUSION: CONNECTION BETWEEN SEXUAL AND REPRODUCTIVE HEALTH

# INTRODUCTION: THE COMPLEXITY OF FERTILITY

Trying to have a baby can feel like a tricky maze—sometimes smooth sailing, sometimes full of surprises and disappointment.

Here's Sarah and David, a couple eager to start a family. At first, they were thrilled about having a baby, and hopeful for the future. But as time passed with no success, they felt uncertain and frustrated. They navigated doctor visits, tried different treatments, and rode a wave of emotions.

Their story is just one piece of the puzzle. Trying to conceive involves understanding our bodies and coping with tough emotions when things don't go as planned. It's a journey with highs and lows.

But amid the challenges, there's hope. Each hurdle makes us stronger. It requires bravery, resilience, and belief in a positive outcome.

So, let's stay positive and open-hearted on this journey. Despite its complexities, there's always a chance for something wonderful to happen.

# CHAPTER ONE: THE BIOLOGICAL CLOCK: UNDERSTANDING FEMALE REPRODUCTIVE AGING

The Biological Clock: Understanding Female Reproductive Aging is a topic that explores the deep connection between a woman's ability to have children and the passing of time. From the moment a baby girl is born, her ovaries contain a limited number of immature egg cells, known as primordial follicles. This ovarian reserve is a precious treasure that decreases with every menstrual cycle, gradually leading to a decline in fertility as a woman approaches her late 30s and early 40s.

Picture a grand opera house, where the ovaries act as the stage, and the follicles are the performers. In the early adult years, the curtain rises on a vibrant show, with numerous follicles vying for their chance to mature and potentially be fertilized. However, as the years go by, the cast grows smaller, and the performances become less frequent.

The concept of the biological clock is deeply rooted in the intricate interplay between hormones and ovarian function. As a woman nears her late 30s, the quality and quantity of her remaining eggs begin to diminish, making it increasingly challenging to conceive naturally. This biological reality showcases the remarkable complexity of the human reproductive system and serves as a gentle reminder that fertility is fleeting.

It's crucial to understand that the biological clock ticks at a unique pace for each woman, influenced by a variety of factors, including genetics, overall health, and lifestyle choices. While some women may experience a gradual decline in fertility, others may face a more abrupt transition, highlighting the importance of open communication with healthcare providers and informed decision-making.

Yet, the biological clock is not merely a harbinger of limitations; it is also a catalyst for empowerment and informed choices. With advancements in reproductive technology, such as in vitro fertilization (IVF) and egg freezing, women now have more options than ever before to preserve their fertility and plan their families according to their unique circumstances and aspirations.

Ultimately, understanding the biological clock is not about instilling fear or imposing societal pressures; rather, it is about embracing the profound beauty and complexity of the female reproductive journey. By acknowledging this natural phenomenon, women can make informed decisions, seek timely medical guidance, and embrace the multifaceted roles they may choose to play throughout their lives – as mothers, professionals, or both.

In a world that often glorifies youth and dismisses the wisdom of age, the biological clock serves as a gentle reminder to cherish the present, plan for the future, and celebrate the extraordinary resilience of the human spirit.

# CHAPTER TWO: FERTILITY TREATMENTS: OPTIONS, SUCCESS RATES, AND CONSIDERATIONS

In a world where the biological clock ticks with relentless precision, these treatments offer a glimmer of hope, a chance to defy the boundaries of nature and embrace the profound joy of parenthood.

Imagine a young couple, Sarah and Michael, who have walked the winding paths of life together, their love a steadfast anchor amidst life's storms. Yet, despite their unwavering devotion, the journey to parenthood has proven arduous, their dreams of cradling a child in their arms seemingly out of reach. It is in this moment of uncertainty that the possibilities of fertility treatments beckon, offering a beacon of hope in the darkness.

The realm of fertility treatments is a vast and ever-evolving landscape, with options ranging from intrauterine insemination (IUI) to the more complex in vitro fertilization (IVF) and intracytoplasmic sperm injection (ICSI). Each option presents its unique characteristics, success rates, and considerations, requiring a delicate balance of medical expertise, emotional resilience, and financial readiness.

IUI, a relatively straightforward procedure, involves placing sperm directly into the uterus during ovulation, offering a gentle nudge towards conception. For couples grappling with mild fertility issues, this approach can yield success rates of up to 20% per cycle, a glimmer of hope that ignites the heart.

For those facing more complex challenges, IVF emerges as a beacon of possibility. In this intricate process, eggs are retrieved from the woman's ovaries and fertilized with sperm in a laboratory setting, creating embryos that are then transferred into the uterus. With success rates ranging from 20% to 35% per cycle, depending on various factors such as age and the cause of infertility, IVF has opened the doors to parenthood for countless individuals and couples.

Yet, within the tapestry of fertility treatments lies another thread – the heartwarming tale of Sarah and Michael. After navigating the intricate maze of options, they decide to embark on the IVF journey, a decision born of unwavering love and steadfast determination. The road is not without its challenges, but each obstacle is met with resilience and hope, fueled by the dream of holding their precious child in their arms.

As the cycle unfolds, Sarah's body responds favorably to the medications and a cluster of viable eggs is retrieved, each one a tiny miracle waiting to be nurtured. In the sterile confines of the laboratory, these eggs are expertly fertilized, and the most promising embryos are carefully selected for transfer.

The transfer day arrives, and Sarah and Michael hold their breath as the embryos are gently introduced into the nurturing embrace of Sarah's womb. In that moment, their dreams, their prayers, and their unwavering love coalesce, creating a tapestry of hope that transcends the boundaries of science.

Weeks pass, each day filled with a delicate blend of anticipation and trepidation, until finally, the news they have longed for is revealed – a positive pregnancy test, a testament to the power of perseverance and the indomitable spirit of love.

As Sarah's belly swells with the miracle of life, she and Michael are reminded that fertility treatments are not merely medical procedures but portals to profound joy, a testament to the resilience of the human spirit and the boundless capacity for love to conquer even the most formidable of obstacles.

# CHAPTER THREE: BEYOND CONCEPTION: THE JOURNEY OF PREGNANCY AND PARENTHOOD

Pregnancy and parenthood are transformative experiences that bring immense joy, along with their fair share of challenges and opportunities for growth. It all starts with the amazing moment of conception, when a sperm fertilizes an egg, leading to the formation of a tiny embryo that finds its home in the mother's womb.

As the pregnancy progresses, the mother's body undergoes incredible changes. Hormones flood her system, nurturing and safeguarding the developing baby. Her belly expands, serving as a visible reminder of the life growing inside her. From the first gentle flutters to the stronger kicks and hiccups, the expectant mother forms a deep bond with her unborn child.

The father also plays a crucial role in this journey, providing support and sharing in the excitement. He attends prenatal appointments with the mother and bonds with the baby through touch and conversation. Together, they make decisions about the birth plan, parenting approach, and creating a nurturing environment for their child.

Throughout the nine months, expectant parents experience a range of emotions and physical changes. They may deal with nausea, fatigue, and mood swings, all while marveling at the miracle unfolding within them. Anticipation builds as they prepare for the arrival of their little one.

Labor and delivery mark the climax of this journey. Contractions signal the onset of labor, bringing the baby closer to taking their first breath. The mother draws on her inner strength during labor, guided by the support of her partner and medical team. Finally, the baby is born, filling the room with cries of life and a flood of overwhelming love.

Parenthood officially begins at that moment, as exhausted but overjoyed parents hold their newborn. The sleepless nights, diaper changes, and round-the-clock feedings become the new norm, punctuated by moments of pure joy as they witness their child's first smile and steps.

Beyond the challenges, parenthood offers unparalleled fulfillment and joy. As children grow, parents witness their unique personalities emerge, guiding and nurturing them along the way. With each milestone achieved and obstacle overcome, the journey of parenthood unfolds, shaping the lives of both parent and child.

The journey of pregnancy and parenthood is an extraordinary adventure, showcasing the resilience of the human body and the boundless capacity for love. Embracing the highs and lows, parents embark on a lifelong journey with their child, filled with boundless love, growth, and endless possibilities.

# CHAPTER FOUR: FERTILITY PRESERVATION: PLANNING FOR THE FUTURE

Fertility preservation is super important for folks who want to plan for having kids. Whether it's because of health issues, getting older, or just personal choice, saving your fertility gives you the chance to have kids later on when you're ready.

Imagine you get a scary diagnosis or have to do a treatment that might mess with your ability to have kids. In those tough times, fertility preservation can be a real lifesaver. It lets you freeze your eggs, sperm, or embryos so you can use them later when you want to start a family.

For women, freezing eggs has become popular. As more women wait longer to have kids for school or work, freezing eggs lets them save their chance to have babies. By freezing eggs when they're young and healthy, women up their odds of getting pregnant down the road.

Men can benefit too from freezing sperm. This is especially helpful if they're getting treatments like chemo or radiation that could mess with their sperm. With frozen sperm, they can still have a shot at being parents even after tough treatments.

But it's not just for medical stuff. Some people want to wait on having kids for their reasons, like wanting to focus on their careers. Freezing eggs, sperm, or embryos lets them protect their chances of having a family later on, even as they get older.

Now, freezing your fertility doesn't guarantee you'll have kids later. But it boosts your chances. And thanks to better technology, these methods are getting easier and more effective, which gives hope to people who thought they might not have options before.

If you're thinking about freezing your fertility, it's smart to talk to experts. They can walk you through the process, check out your situation, and suggest the best plan based on your goals and health.

In the end, fertility preservation is all about giving people control over when they have kids. By taking action now, you're making sure that having a family is still possible, no matter what life throws your way. It's like investing in your future family, bringing peace of mind and the

chance to make your dream of being a
parent come true.

# CHAPTER FIVE: THE PSYCHOLOGICAL IMPACT: NAVIGATING EMOTIONAL CHALLENGES

Preserving your fertility isn't just about the physical stuff; it's a wild ride of emotions that can mess with your head. Dealing with the ups and downs of this journey takes guts, help from others, and understanding the complicated feelings that pop up.

Imagine the whirlwind of emotions when you realize your ability to have kids might be in jeopardy. It's scary, sad, and feels like you've lost something big. The idea of not being able to have a baby naturally can hit hard and make it tough to handle all those feelings.

For some, deciding to save their fertility comes after a big health scare, like cancer or a serious illness. This adds even more stress on top of worrying about your health. Feeling anxious, mad, and like you've lost control is common, making it even harder to deal with the whole fertility thing.

Even if you're freezing your fertility for reasons like work or just personal choice, it's still a big emotional deal. There's pressure from society, the fear of missing out on the "right" time to have kids, and not knowing what's coming next can be a lot to handle.

When dealing with all these emotions, taking care of yourself and leaning on your support system is key. Having understanding people around who listen and care can help you get through it.

Remember, it's normal to feel sad, mad, or anxious during this process. Letting yourself feel those emotions without judging can be a big step in feeling better.

Getting help from a pro therapist who knows about fertility stuff can also be a game-changer. They can give you tools to cope, help you sort through your feelings, and give you a safe space to discuss your worries without feeling judged.

Ultimately, dealing with the emotional side of fertility preservation means being kind to yourself, getting support, and reaching out for help when you need it. By facing these challenges and getting the help you need, you can come out stronger and more resilient on the other side.

# CONCLUSION: CONNECTION BETWEEN SEXUAL AND REPRODUCTIVE HEALTH

In the field of medicine, sexual and reproductive health are intimately related. Let's break it down:

Sexual health is about feeling good physically, emotionally, mentally, and socially about your sexuality. It's having safe, respectful sexual experiences without feeling pressured or facing violence.

Reproductive health focuses on your reproductive system's well-being. It includes choosing when to have kids and taking care of your body during pregnancy.

It's super important for human rights and treating everyone fairly, ensuring communities can thrive. Even the United Nations aims to give everyone access to top-notch reproductive healthcare.

The goal is to keep individuals, couples, and families happy and healthy, no matter who they are. It's not just about making babies; it's also about how people connect, feel, and think about sex and relationships.

Ensuring women have the same rights as men is a big part of this. It's about empowering everyone to make informed choices about their bodies and get quality healthcare.

Empowering Choices for Reproductive Health

Deciding about your reproductive health is a big deal. Whether you're saving your fertility for later or dealing with all the ups and downs, it's about feeling powerful.

Choosing to freeze your eggs, sperm, or embryos puts you in control of your family plans down the road. It's like having a safety net, so you can still have kids no matter what happens.

And when you're dealing with all the emotions, it's okay to feel everything. Having supportive people around and getting help from professionals can help.

So, whether you're facing a tough health problem, waiting to have kids for your reasons, or want to be proactive, remember you've

got options. And by making those choices, you're taking control of your story, giving yourself the power to create the future you want.

www.ingramcontent.com/pod-product-compliance
Lightning Source LLC
Chambersburg PA
CBHW072342270726
48659CB00023B/2311